Date Due

CAT. NO. 23 233   PRINTED IN U.S.A.

MEDICINE
in
art

Fine Art Books for Young People

AMERICAN HISTORY *in Art*
The BIRD *in Art*
The BLACK MAN *in Art*
The CAT *in Art*
CIRCUSES *and* FAIRS *in Art*
The CITY *in Art*
DEMONS *and* BEASTS *in Art*
FARMS *and* FARMERS *in Art*
The HORSE *in Art*
KINGS *and* QUEENS *in Art*
MEDICINE *in Art*
MUSICAL INSTRUMENTS *in Art*
The SELF-PORTRAIT *in Art*
The SHIP *and the* SEA *in Art*
SPORTS *and* GAMES *in Art*
The WARRIOR *in Art*
The WORKER *in Art*
The OLD TESTAMENT *in Art*
The NEW TESTAMENT *in Art*

*We specialize in producing quality
books for young people. For a complete list please write*

LERNER PUBLICATIONS COMPANY
241 First Avenue North, Minneapolis, Minnesota 55401

MEDICINE
in
art

By Rena Neumann Coen, Ph.D. Designed by Patricia Koskey ■ Lerner Publications Company, Minneapolis, Minn.

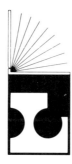

Second Printing 1971

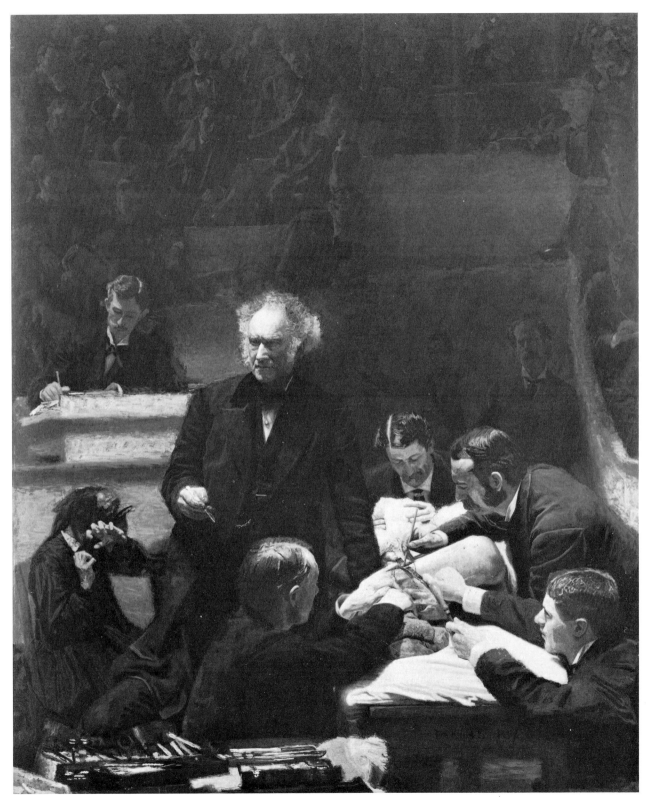

The Gross Clinic (1875), by Thomas Eakins (1844-1916); Jefferson Medical College, Philadelphia; photographed by The Philadelphia Museum of Art.

Contents

Introduction

Birth, life, death, good health and bad are the essence of the human experience. Artists, being human too, have shown a natural interest in these experiences and have recorded in painting and sculpture the physical condition of man.

As long as there have been sickness, disease, or injury, there have also been attempts at cures. In ancient times, as well as in primitive societies, cure was believed to be effected through magic, and the physician was regarded either as a magician or as a being endowed with divine powers. Today, medicine is practiced as a science, but some of the medicines we now use were discovered and first used by very primitive healers.

From ancient times too, there were laws regulating the practice of those who attempted to cure the sick. The *stele*, or stone monument, of Hammurabi, who was King of Babylon around 1900 B.C., bears such a code of laws on its surface. Among a list of other legal regulations, it deals with the fees that may be charged for successful medical treatment and the punishment to be given those who attempt a cure but instead cause further injury. Above the inscription the king is shown standing in prayer before the sun-god Shamash, "Lord of Justice and Law Giver." The god is seated on a throne, wearing a crown and holding a ring and a rod whose symbolic meaning is unknown. The figures confront each other in the stiff, formal attitudes that match the religious significance of the scene.

As time went on, other artists illustrated other aspects of sickness and health, of medicines and those who administer them, and of the buildings and hospitals where the sick were cared for. Though attitudes toward disease and the practice of medicine have changed greatly since the days of Hammurabi, the artist's fascination with the subject has remained as strong as ever. It is a subject that has inspired innumerable works of art, from the beginning of history to the present day. Only a small sample of these can be included in this book on medicine in art.

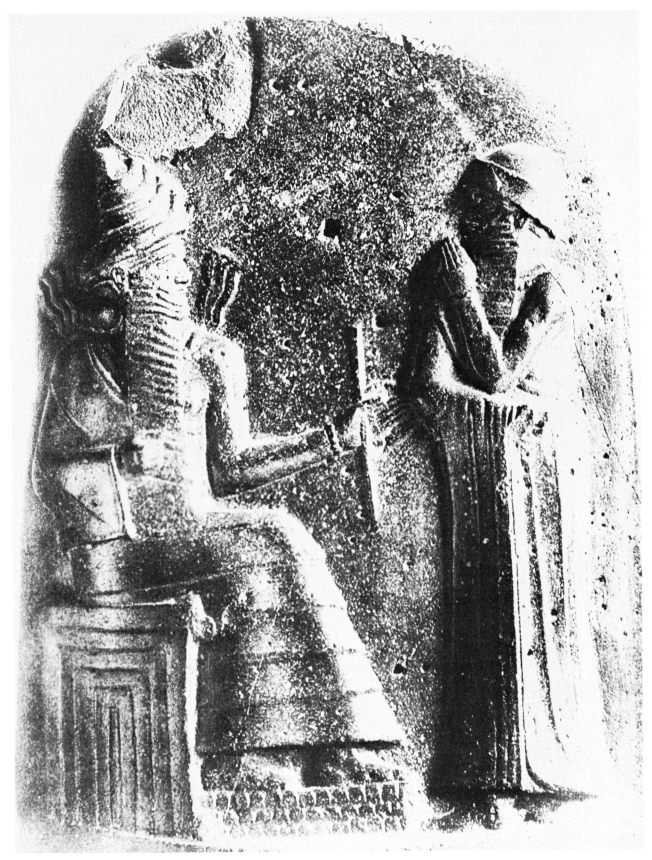

Babylonian stele of Hammurabi receiving law code from the sun god (19th century B.C.); Louvre, Paris; University Prints, Boston.

Birth, Life, Death

The most important events in human existence take place without our being fully aware of them. Man does not remember his birth, he is not consciously aware of his life (unless it is threatened), and oblivion follows the moment of death.

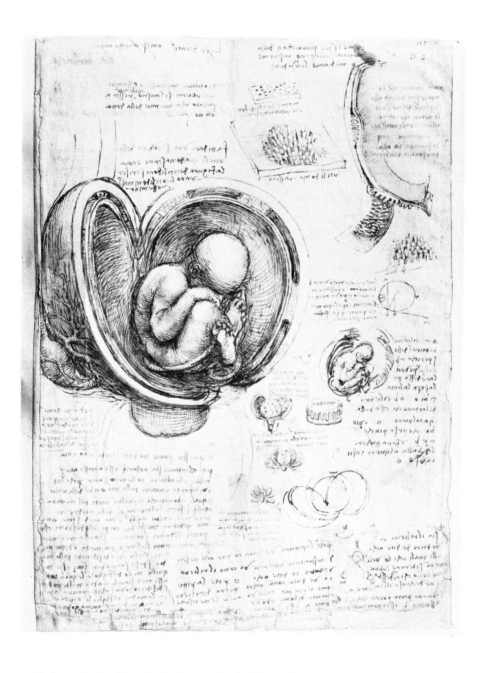

Embryo in the Womb, by Leonardo da Vinci (1452-1519); Royal Collection, Windsor Castle, Berkshire; reproduced by gracious permission of Her Majesty Queen Elizabeth II.

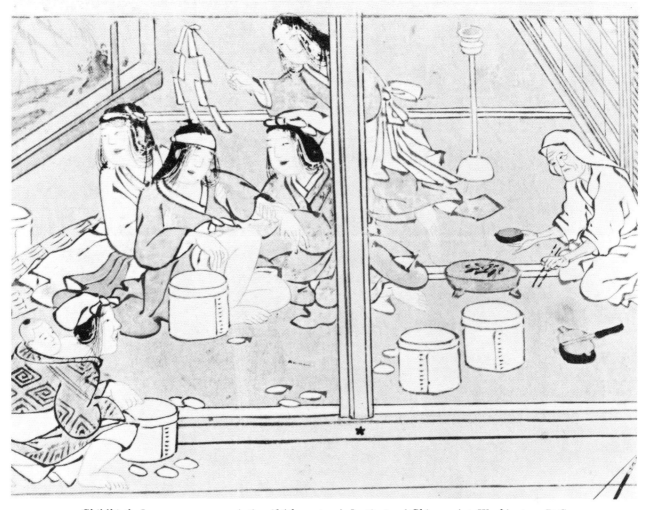

Childbirth, Japanese screen painting (14th century); Institute of Chinese Art, Washington, D.C.

Birth comes after the development of the embryo in its mother's womb. Leonardo da Vinci's (lay-oh-NAR-doh da VIN-chee) pen drawing of an embryo in the womb is one of the many beautiful anatomical studies he drew. An artist of the Italian Renaissance, Leonardo reflected in his drawings the age's re-awakened curiosity in nature and in man. This drawing includes his notations (written backwards in mirror- writing) on the anatomy of the embryo. The same kind of careful study lay behind the artist's life-like representations of the human body in his finished paintings. The embryo in the womb is carefully drawn in a beautiful, fluid hand that recorded accurately the appearance of the unborn child.

Childbirth itself has been more frequently illustrated in primitive and in oriental societies than in the West where reserve and concealment have accompanied this normal human experience. A Japanese screen painting of the 14th century illustrates a woman in childbirth surrounded by the women who attend her. The painting is flat and colorful. The artist, though interested in the event he is portraying, is equally interested in the pattern of color, line, and graceful form created by his painting.

10

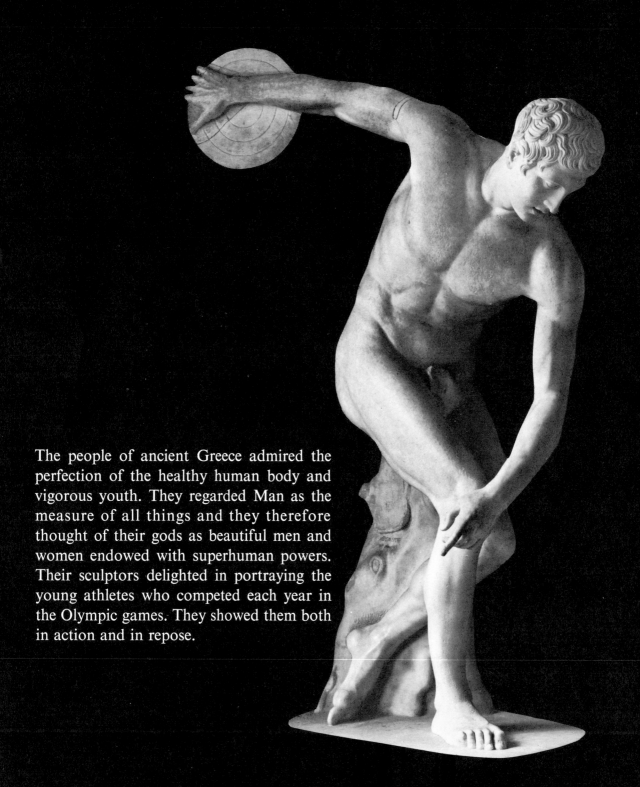

The people of ancient Greece admired the perfection of the healthy human body and vigorous youth. They regarded Man as the measure of all things and they therefore thought of their gods as beautiful men and women endowed with superhuman powers. Their sculptors delighted in portraying the young athletes who competed each year in the Olympic games. They showed them both in action and in repose.

Discobolus (450 B.C.), by Myron (fifth century B.C.); Vatican Museum, Rome; Alinari, Art Reference Bureau.

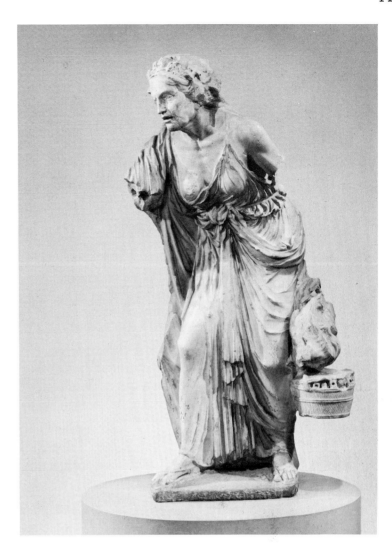

Old Market Woman (second century B.C.);
The Metropolitan Museum of Art, New
York; Rogers Fund, 1909.

Myron, an Athenian sculptor of the fifth century B.C., was the creator of the *Discobolus* (Discus Thrower) which was carved around 450 B.C. at the height of the golden age of Greek art. Though the original sculpture is lost, enough ancient copies exist to give us a good idea of what Myron's *Discobolus* looked like. The young athlete is shown just before he throws the flat but heavy discus. His body is coiled like a tightly-wound spring. In a moment it will spin round with the full force of suddenly released energy — and the discus will fly toward the distant target. Yet this is more than a study of physical force and controlled energy. If you look at the picture carefully, you will see that the artist has created a beautiful harmony between the mass of the carved marble and the voids, or empty spaces, that surround it. This balance of form and space, of tension and release, is the measure of truly great sculpture.

It was not until the later years of Greek civilization that sculptors began to portray the less ideal aspects of human existence — sickness, old age, and death. An unknown sculptor of the second century B.C. carved a marble statue of an *Old Market Woman*. Bent and weary, leaning heavily on a staff that has now disappeared, the old woman hobbles to market with her basket of produce. Her flesh and her spirit sag with the weight of years and the disappointments that life has brought her.

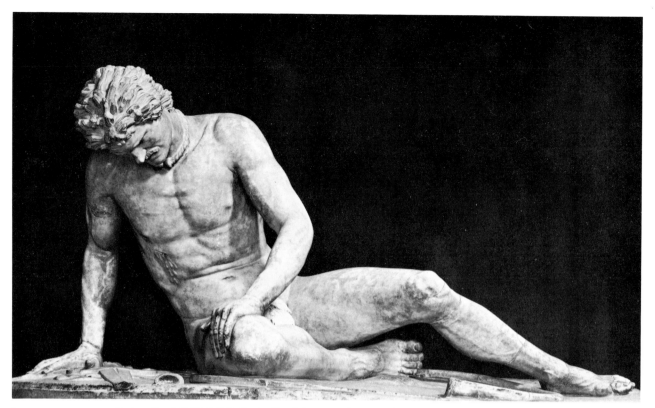

Dying Gaul (230 B.C.); Capitoline Museum, Rome; Alinari, Art Reference Bureau.

Death too was depicted by the later Greeks whose culture had spread far beyond the confines of Greece itself. The *Dying Gaul*, dating from around 230 B.C., is a Roman copy of a Greek original. This is no longer the ideal portrait of Myron's *Discobolus* whose features are a generalized summary of young manhood. This is rather a truthful study of a real person, a Gaul, who has been defeated in battle. Pride, suffering, and endurance are reflected in his attitude as the moment of death approaches. Round his neck he wears a torque, the twisted necklace worn by the Gauls. He has the shaggy hair of a barbarian yet the Greek sculptor was not contemptuous of him. He shows the dying Gaul as a hero, a brave warrior, endowed at the moment of death with nobility and grandeur.

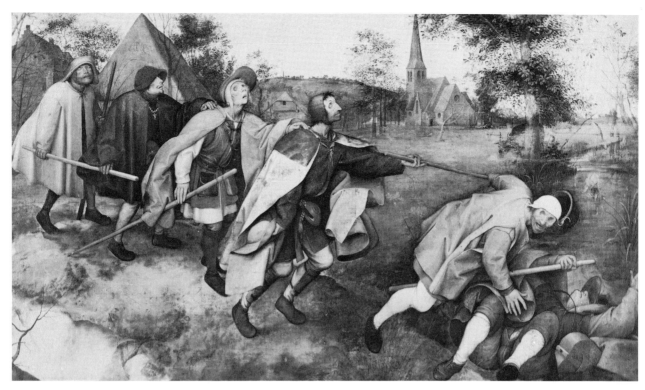

The Parable of the Blind Men, by Peter Brueghel the Elder (1525-1659);
Museum of Naples; Alinari, Art Reference Bureau.

The Blind, the Lame, the Halt

Peter Brueghel the Elder (BREW-gul), a Dutch artist of the 16th century, illustrated *The Parable of the Blind Men* in the painting shown here. It is hard to tell whether Brueghel felt sorry for the blind men or not. They are pathetic as well as grotesque. Guided only by their sense of touch, they stumble through a lovely landscape which they cannot see. Their leader tumbles into a ditch, and the blind men, sightless and helpless, will soon follow him. But in the background all is serene. Feathery trees suggest an early spring, a winding stream leads our eye into a peaceful meadow, and an old church nestles into the distant hills.

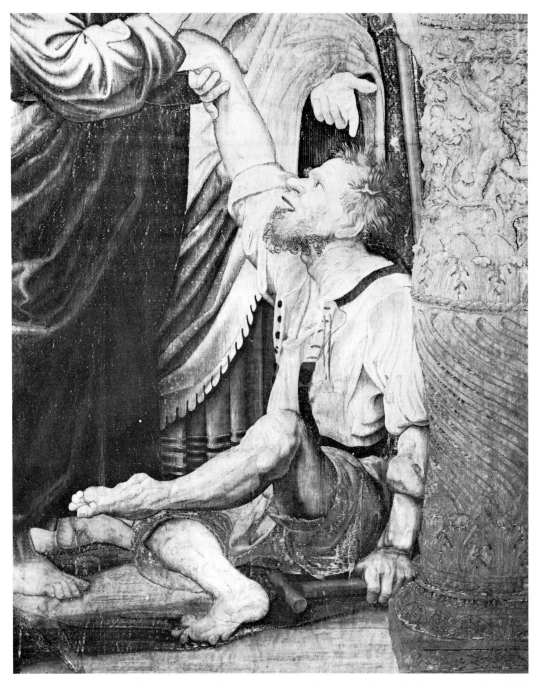

The Healing of the Cripple, detail from the tapestry of a Miraculous Cure, by Raphael (1483-1520); Vatican Museum, Rome; Alinari, Art Reference Bureau.

The Healing of the Cripple is a detail from a tapestry in the Vatican Palace in Rome. A tapestry is a picture woven in colored wool or silk and wool. The *cartoon*, or sketch, for this tapestry was drawn by the great Italian Renaissance painter, Raphael (RAH-fa-ell).

Obviously he had observed crippled men very closely. The unfortunate man's twisted limbs are carefully drawn and even the little wheeled platform on which he propelled himself is shown. The cripple's face is lit up with joy at the miraculous cure that, according to the biblical story, is about to occur.

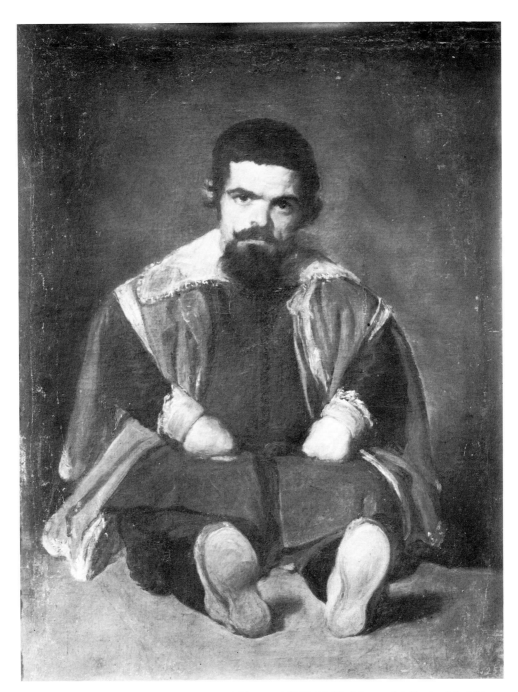

Don Sebastian de Mora, by Diego Velásquez (1599-1660); Museo del Prado, Madrid.

A cripple of a different sort is shown in Velásquez's *Don Sebastian de Mora*. Diego Velásquez (vuh-LAS-kez) was official painter to the Spanish king, Philip IV, whose family and court he painted many times. Don Sebastian was a dwarf whose legs and arms were abnormally small in relation to the rest of his body. Such deformed people were often kept at European courts to provide amusement for the noble ladies and gentlemen who surrounded the king. They were expected to be witty and entertaining and to provide a note of cheer in the stiffly formal atmosphere of the king's court. But the sad-eyed man looking out at us from Velásquez's portrait hardly looks like a cheerful entertainer.

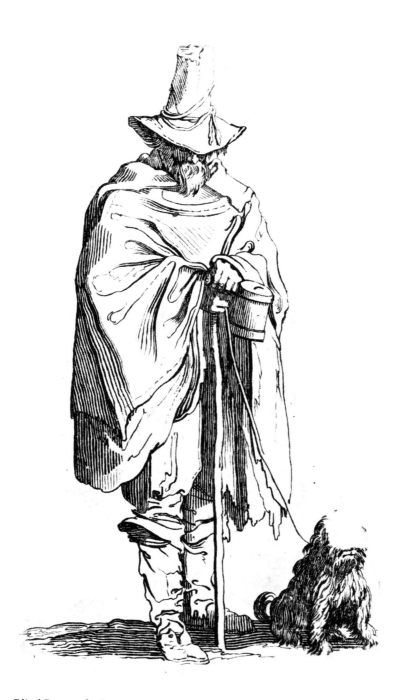

Blind Beggar, by Jacques Callot (1592-1635); Bibliothèque Nationale, Paris; Photograph Giraudon.

In the past, society gave little care to its physically handicapped members. Crippled or blind people often had no choice but to go out on the street with a small cup or box and beg passers for a coin to buy a crust of bread. Jacques Callot (zhahk kah-LOW), a 17th-century French artist, used the outcasts of society — its cripples, beggars, hired soldiers, or wandering actors — to illustrate the life he saw around him. His *Blind Beggar* is wrapped in rags and his own sad thoughts as he holds an alms box out to the world. A little dog is his only protector and companion. There is both deep compassion and an implied criticism of society in this quick ink sketch of a poor and lonely cripple.

Sickness of Body and Mind

Disease as well as physical deformity provided subject matter for artists of different periods and countries. A mother with a sick child, for example, is a universal theme — a human situation that saddens every observer. It is a theme that was illustrated in two totally different ways by Gabriel Metsu in 17th-century Holland and by the Norwegian painter Edvard Munch (moongk) in 20th-century Paris.

Metsu's child lies listlessly in her mother's lap. She may not be feeling very well, but her mother looks so buxom and strong and her home so comfortable that we feel sure she is getting the best of care. Metsu has been careful to arrange the people and objects in the room in a pleasant, balanced composition. The figures have weight and solidity and, despite the sickness of the child, the picture

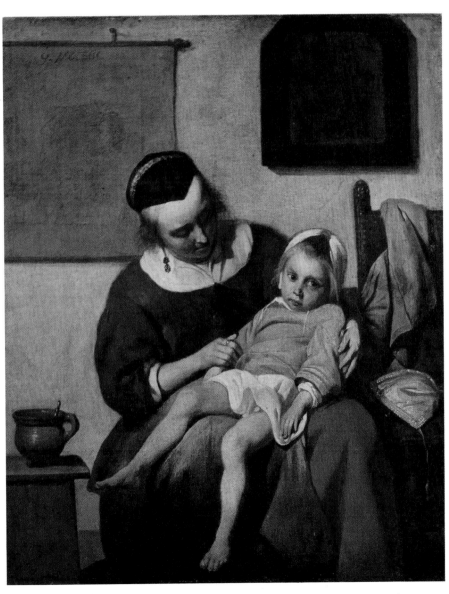

The Sick Child, by Gabriel Metsu (1629-1667); Rijksmuseum, Amsterdam.

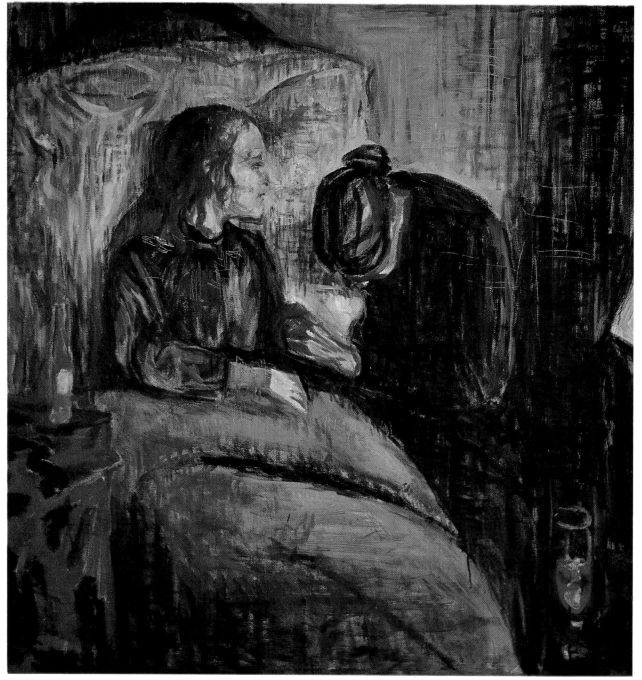

The Sick Child, by Edvard Munch (1863-1944); Municipal Collections, Munch Museum, Oslo.

is not a sad one. Munch's picture, on the other hand, is ominous. It tells us clearly and vividly that illness is not pleasant. With a few bold, slashing brushstrokes that express his deep emotion, this artist depicts a very sick girl, white and worn, propped up in bed with her mother beside her. We are afraid that this girl will not recover and we cannot help sharing the grief of her despairing mother.

Sick adults, as well as children, have often been the subjects of an artist's brush — and occasionally the patients have even been the artists themselves.

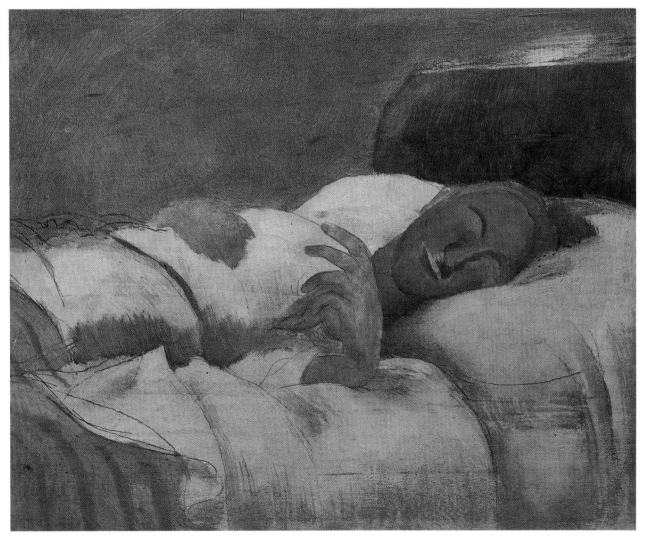

The Sick Man, by Roger de la Fresnaye (1885-1925); Musée National d'Art Moderne, Paris.

A less intense but no less vivid portrayal of illness is *The Sick Man* by Roger de la Fresnaye (ro-zhay du la fray-neh) a French 20th-century artist. With only a few simplified forms and a limited but warm color range, de la Fresnaye managed to suggest the fever that wracks the patient. The swirling lines that indicate the bed sheets and the listless movement of the hand heighten the illusion of the confused state of mind frequently induced by a high fever.

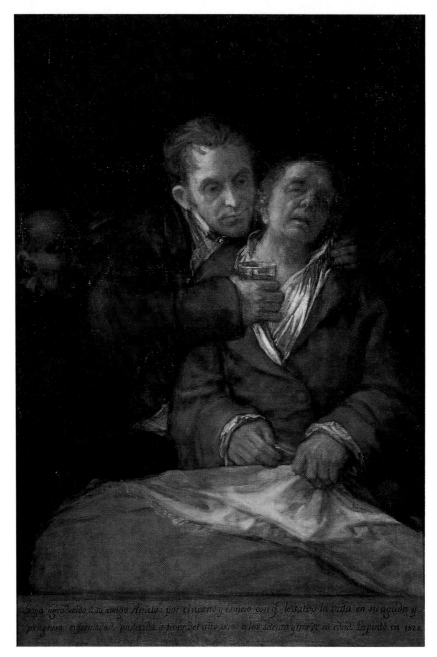

Self-Portrait with Dr. Arrieta (1820) by Francisco Goya (1746-1828); Minneapolis Institute of Arts; Ethel Morrison Van Derlip Fund.

In 1820 the Spanish artist Francisco Goya (GO-yah) painted his *Self-Portrait with Dr. Arrieta*. The artist is shown propped up in bed, leaning on the arm of his friend, Dr. Arrieta, who offers him a glass of medicine to drink. The sick man clutches weakly at the bed sheets for additional support, in a marvellous portrayal of exhaustion and infirmity. The subdued colors, the murky light, and the indistinct faces in the background add to the somber mood of illness and suffering. Goya recovered, however, and the following year inscribed the painting to Dr. Arrieta with these words: "Goya thanks his friend Arrieta for the sureness and care with which he saved his life from serious and dangerous illness suffered at the end of the year 1819 at the age of seventy-three. Painted in 1820."

A very famous painting of a sick man is to be found on an alterpiece painted by the German artist Mathias Grünewald (GRUE-nuh-vahlt) for the Antonite monks of Isenheim. These monks cared for sick people suffering from a disease called *ergotism* or "St. Anthony's Fire." It was caused by eating bread made of moldy or rotten grain and its symptoms included large, painful boils that erupted all over the body. The clinical accuracy with which Grünewald recorded this disease is typical of his interest in reproducing the natural appearance of physical objects. At the same time, it reflects the preoccupation with the horrible that characterized the art of the early 16th century, a period of intellectual and religious upheaval in Europe.

Temptation of St. Anthony, detail from the Crucifixion scene, by Mathias Grünewald (1470/80-1528); Isenheim Altar, Colmar; Photograph Bulloz, Art Reference Bureau.

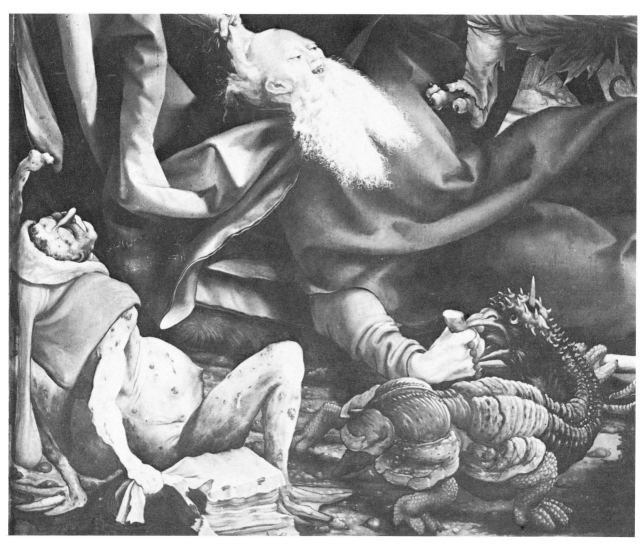

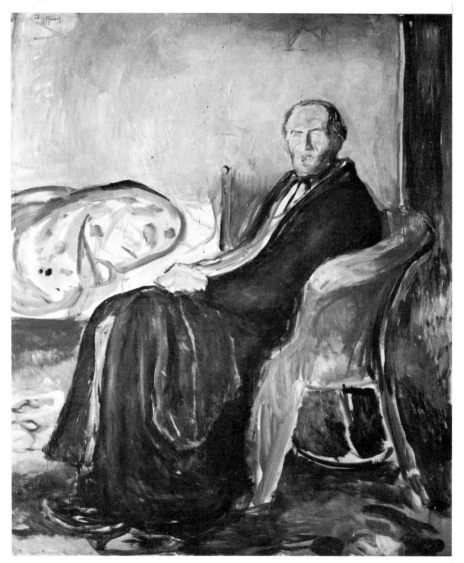

Self-Portrait with Spanish Influenza, by Edvard Munch (1863-1944); National Gallery, Oslo.

Munch, whose *Sick Girl* we have already seen, also painted himself as an invalid. While Goya evoked illness through the portrayal of a weak, pale person propped up in bed with a concerned friend to help him, Munch expresses pain and illness through his bold and heavy brushstrokes. The handling of the paint itself reveals the artist's inmost feelings. This type of painting — called *Expressionism* — is a style that has become identified with a group of early 20th-century painters in Germany and Scandinavia.

Illness, of course, can be mental as well as physical, and modern research points to some sort of connection between the two. *The Mad Assassin* was painted by the 19th-century French painter, Théodore Géricault (zhai-ree-coe). The gaunt face and hollow cheeks, the staring, vacant eyes and unkempt appearance present a clinical study of mental disease. The painting is also a highly dramatic work of art. The drama and the suffering it implies appealed to the taste of the early 19th century. Followers of the Romantic movement in literature and art admired the more unusual and violent aspects of the human and natural environment.

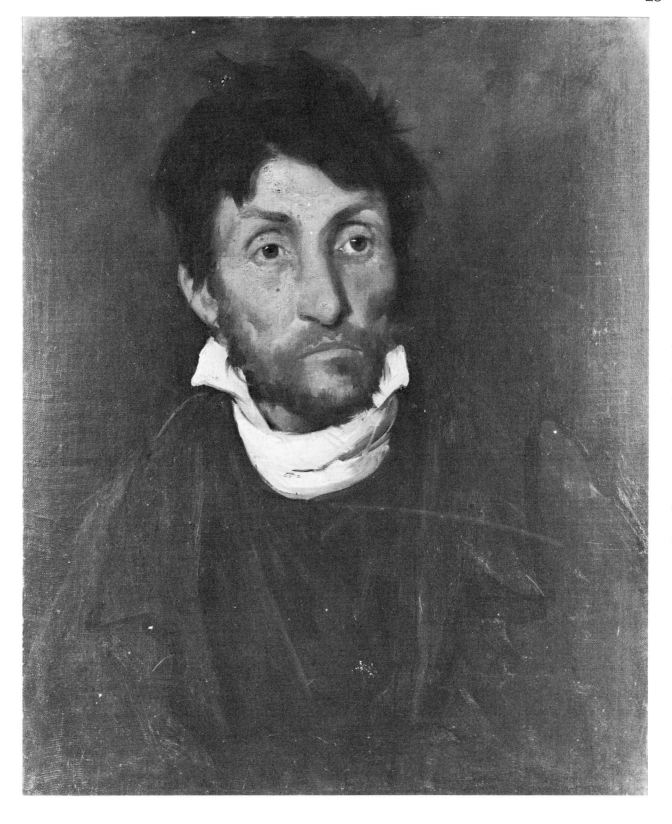

The Mad Assassin, by Théodore Géricault (1791-1824); Musée des Beaux Arts, Gand; Photograph Giraudon.

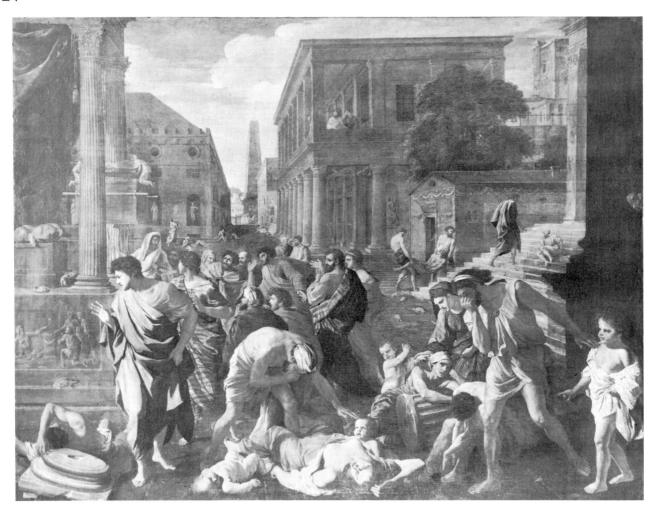

The Philistines Stricken with the Plague, by Nicholas Poussin (1594-1665); Louvre, Paris; Photograph Giraudon.

Before the advent of modern scientific medicine and enlightened public health programs, deadly epidemics wiped out whole cities and destroyed the population of entire countries. Such an epidemic is illustrated in *The Philistines Stricken with the Plague* by Nicolas Poussin (poo-SAN), a French painter of the 17th century. Poussin chose a biblical theme for this dramatic painting but he could as well have illustrated the plagues which swept through Europe in his own century. It is interesting that, amid the corpses and the frightened survivors rushing madly about,

Poussin included a number of large rats in front of a classical temple on the right. The significance of rats as disease carriers was just beginning to be understood during the 17th century.

Poussin's illustration of the plague is a rich and exciting picture done in oil paints on canvas. Its colors are warm and glowing and the drama of the scene is heightened by the concentration of action in the foreground and the stage-set arrangement of the stately buildings in the back.

25

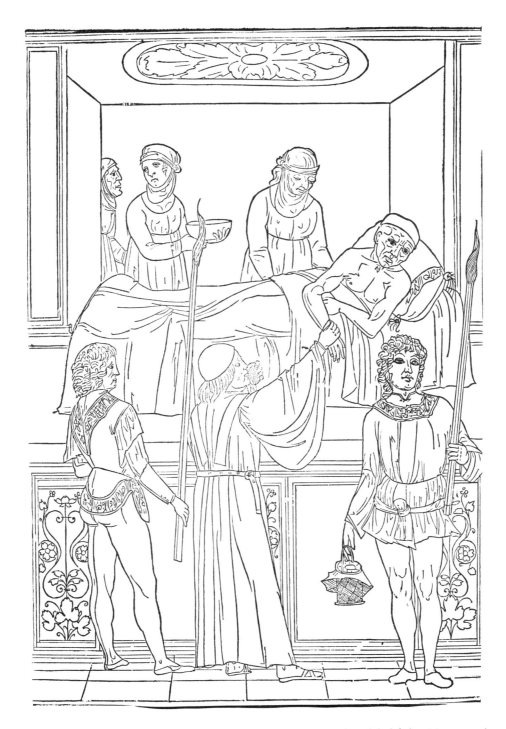

Visit to a Plague Patient, by Gentile Bellini (1429-1507); The Philadelphia Museum of Art; Ars Medica Collection; photograph by A. J. Wyatt, staff photographer.

A much simpler but equally revealing picture of the plague is a line engraving by the Italian 15th-century artist, Gentile Bellini. Called *Visit to a Plague Patient*, it shows a doctor holding a disinfectant-soaked sponge in front of his nose as he feels the patient's pulse. Two attendants hold lighted torches beside him in a further effort to ward off contagion. When preventive medicine and miracle drugs were still unknown, it took both courage and dedication to come to the aid of a patient suffering from the plague.

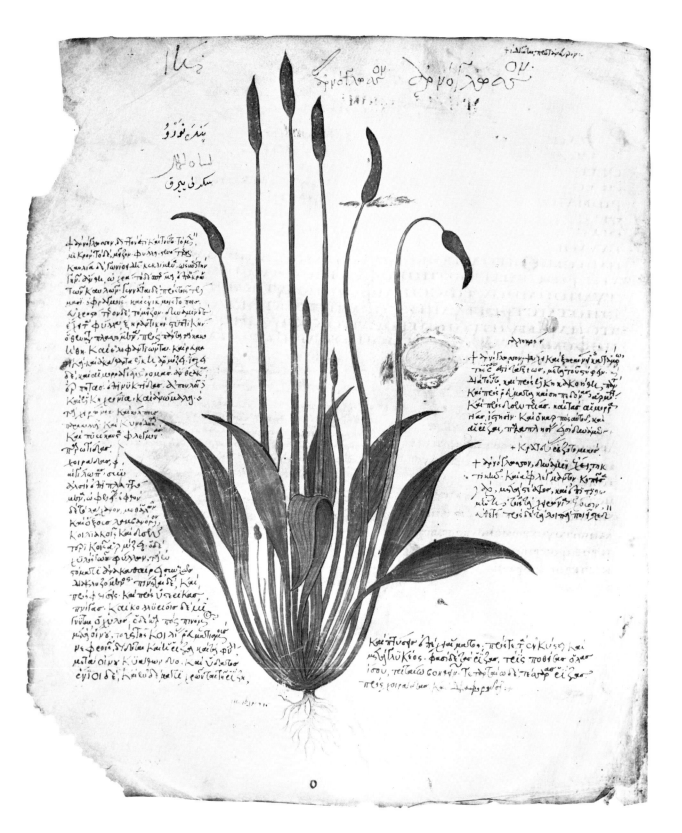

Page of Medical Herbs and Medicinal Recipes from Dioscurides Manuscript of Queen Anisia (sixth century); Austrian National Library, Vienna.

The Cure

Good Medicine and Bad

A familiarity with the healing properties of various herbs and plants goes back to very ancient times. Indeed, many of the brews and herb teas our ancestors made to cure their ailments are recognized by doctors today as effective medicines. The knowledge of these medical plants, gained originally by trial and error, was transmitted to succeeding generations by word of mouth and also in *illuminated*, or illustrated manuscripts.

One such illuminated manuscript dates from as early as the sixth century A.D., or 1400 years ago. The manuscript is a collection of the medical recipes of an ancient Greek physician named Dioscurides who studied medicinal herbs and wrote down what he learned about them. A Greek queen owned this copy of Dioscurides's medical notes and recipes and therefore it is called by her name, *The Manuscript of Queen Anisia*. The plant forms a graceful design, for the artist wanted to please the eye as much as he wanted to be scientifically accurate. The marginal notes written in Greek, and those above in Arabic, describe the medical properties of this plant; they form a pleasant frame for its curling leaves and long, graceful stems.

Sometimes magic chants accompanied the preparation of a medicinal brew. The American Indians entrusted the task of healing to medicine men who were special members of the tribe. These medicine men often had an elementary knowledge of bonesetting and a more profound knowledge of medicinal plants and herbs. But they invoked divine help through special charms and rituals to help them in their work.

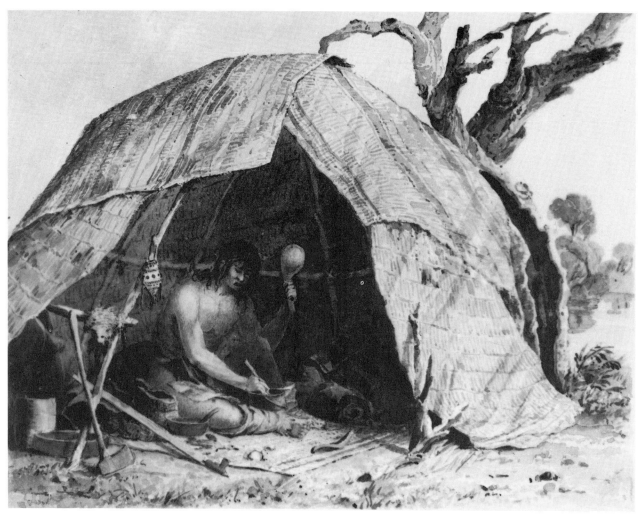

Indian Doctor Concocting a Pot of Medicine, by Seth Eastman (1808-1875); James Jerome Hill Reference Library, St. Paul.

Seth Eastman, an American army officer, sketched many watercolors of Indian life in the western territories. Eastman was Commandant of the frontier outpost of Fort Snelling in the Minnesota territory during the 1840's. One of his watercolors is *Indian Doctor Concocting a Pot of Medicine.* The doctor, or medicine man, sits in a wigwam, shaking a gourd rattle and uttering a magic formula as he stirs the brew in the pot. If the medicine itself didn't work, the patient's faith in its effectiveness often did.

Most medicines in the past tasted worse than they do today because no one had learned how to disguise their bitter taste. Adriaen Brouwer painted *The Bitter Draught*, an amusing picture of a patient swallowing, with some difficulty, a bad-tasting medicine. Brouwer, a Flemish painter of the 17th century, liked to paint the ordinary people he saw around him. He had no pretensions to elegance or refinement. If his characters seem crude and noisy, they nevertheless reflect the artist's own enjoyment of life, and a real sympathy for his fellow man.

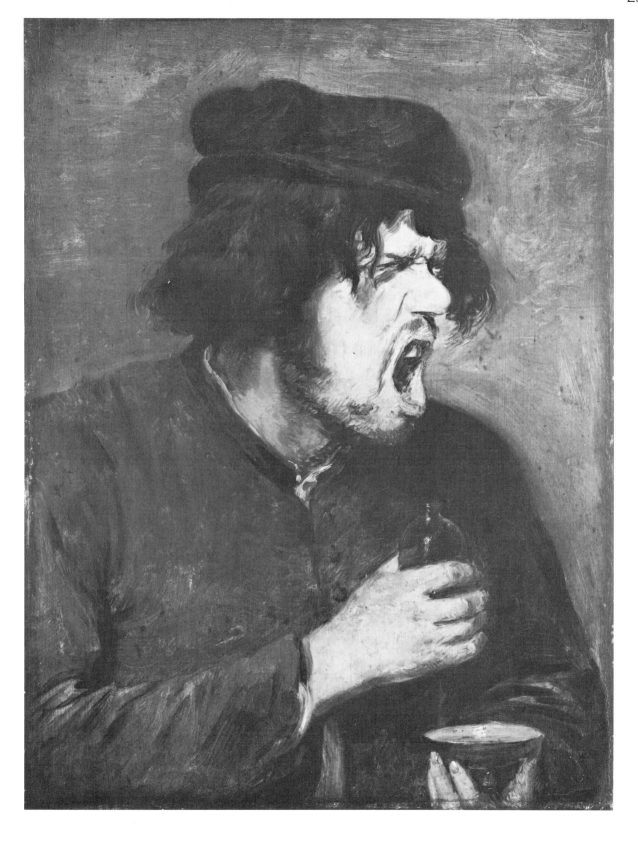

The Bitter Draught, by Adriaen Brouwer (1605-1638); Stadel Institute, Frankfurt.

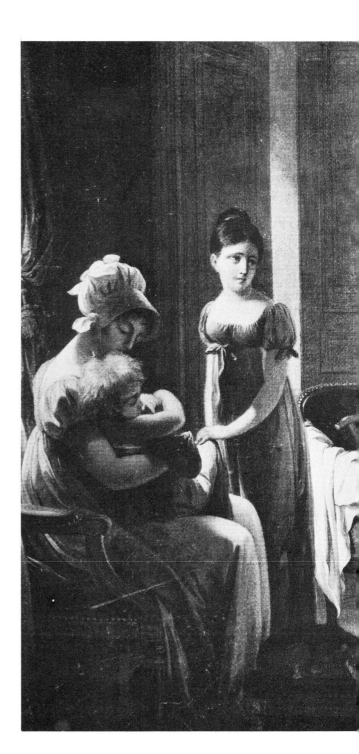

Right: The Vaccination, by Louis Boilly (1761-1845); Collection of Count du Bourg de Bozas; Les Productions de Paris.

The practice of preventive medicine provided a theme for some artists. One of the most important discoveries in preventive medicine was made in 1796, when Edward Jenner, an English doctor, discovered the smallpox vaccine. By the beginning of the 19th century the use of preventive vaccination had spread rapidly throughout Europe and America. Indeed, as early as 1804, President Thomas Jefferson directed the explorers Lewis and Clark to carry a "kine box," or smallpox vaccination kit, with them on their journey through the newly purchased Louisiana territory.

In Europe, at about the same time, the French artist Louis Boilly (bwa-yee) painted *The Vaccination.* Boilly's picture suggests that this new form of preventive medicine had become generally accepted by the early 19th century. In a room bathed in a soft, white light, an old doctor sits and vaccinates a number of children as their mothers and one father look on. The figures are composed in a graceful, harmonious group. They have a quiet dignity that is quite different from Adriaen Brouwer's down-to-earth approach.

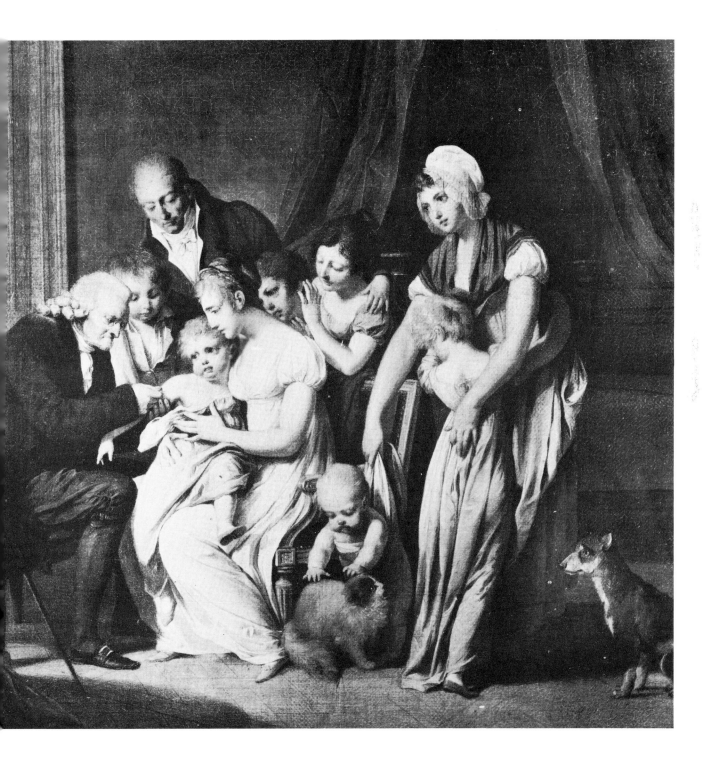

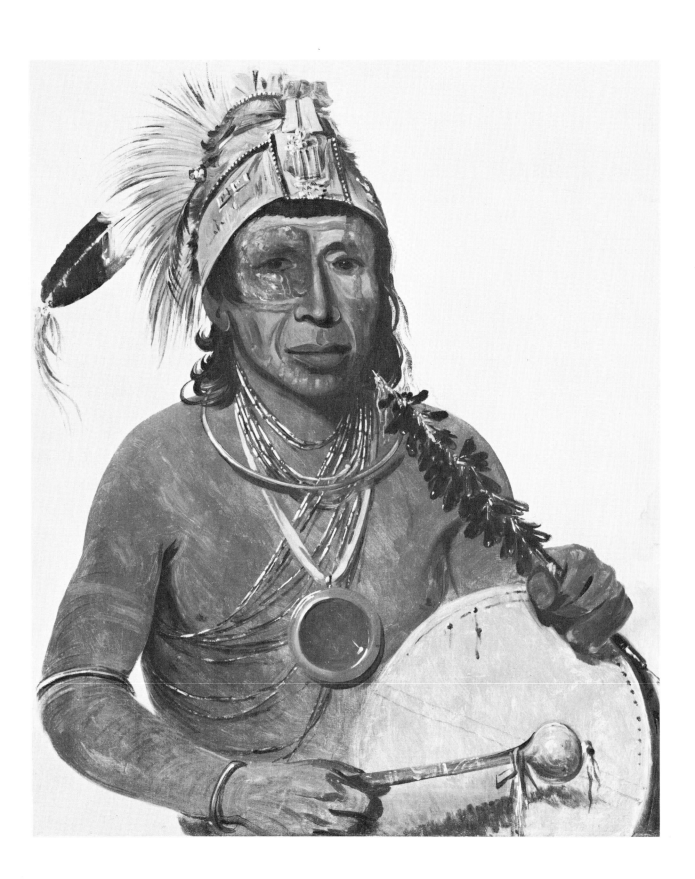

Quacks and Medicine Men

Blue Medicine, or Tah-to-wah-kon-da-pee, was a famous American Indian medicine man. George Catlin, who travelled west and lived among the Indians, painted a portrait of Blue Medicine beating on a medicine drum made of deerskins and shaking a mystery rattle made of antelope hoofs. His face is painted with broad stripes according to the custom of his people. Beads, bracelets, and feather headdress indicate his superior position in the tribe. Blue Medicine occasionally obtained professional tips and even drugs from a white doctor stationed at a frontier post nearby. The white man, however, brought disease as well as medicine to the Indians. Five years after George Catlin had stayed with them, the Mandan tribe of North Dakota was almost completely wiped out by an epidemic of smallpox which had been unknown to them before the arrival of the white man.

Seth Eastman, whose *Indian Doctor Concocting a Pot of Medicine* we have already seen, also painted *Medicine Dance of the Dakota Indians*. The dancers were members of the Medicine Society to which women as well as men could belong. This dance was

Left: Blue Medicine (1835), by George Catlin (1796-1872); National Collection of Fine Arts, Smithsonian Institution, Washington, D.C.

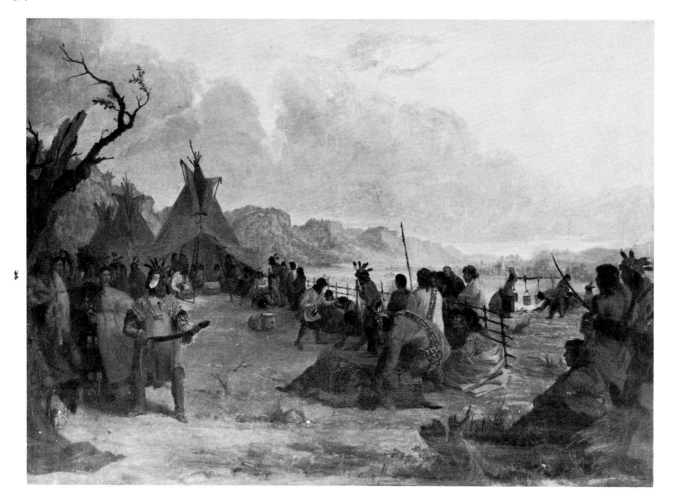

Medicine Dance of the Dakota Indians, by Seth Eastman (1808-1875); Peabody Museum, Harvard University, Cambridge.

actually part of the initiation rite through which new members were accepted into this most sought-after society. It is performed in the open air before a tepee. A soft, atmospheric light bathes the distant bluffs in a misty veil. As in all Eastman paintings, the Indians seem very much a part of their environment. The accuracy with which Eastman recorded the life of the Plains Indians places him in the forefront of Indian historians as well as artists.

The practice of medicine by magicians, medicine men, or charlatans was not confined to the New World or to primitive societies. In Europe, and in America too, people who were not really doctors practiced what might be called at best a kind of pseudo-medicine or at worst, downright fakery.

In *The Visit to the Quack Doctor* William Hogarth presents a fierce caricature of such a charlatan in 18th-century London. Busily polishing his spectacles with a dirty handkerchief, the quack doctor confronts his frightened patient and the young nobleman who brings her. The "doctor's" assistant is a young, richly dressed woman who looks as disagreeable as the quack doctor himself. Skulls, skeletons, dirty instruments, and dusty books are scattered through the room to lend an air of learning and medical competence. This attack on false and dangerous medicine combines realism with savage satire.

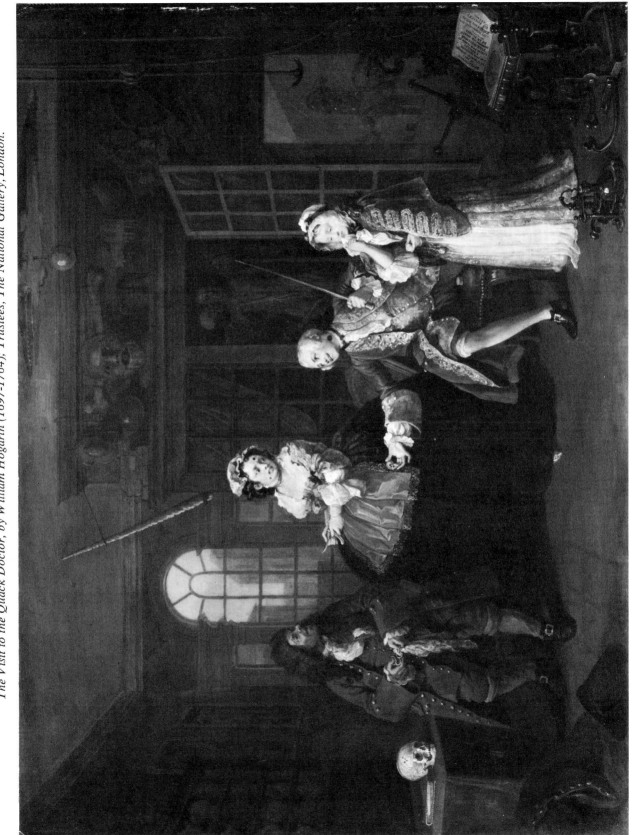

The Visit to the Quack Doctor, by William Hogarth (1697-1764); Trustees, The National Gallery, London.

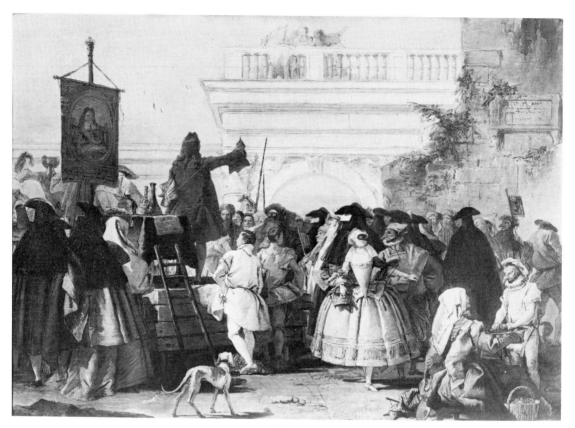

The Charlatan, by Giovanni Battista Tiepolo (1698-1770); Gallery of the Papadopoli Palace, Venice; Alinari, Art Reference Bureau.

In a lighter vein, but no less critical, is Giovanni Battista Tiepolo's (tee-AY-poh-loh) painting, *The Charlatan.* Tiepolo was a Venetian contemporary of Hogarth, and his painting demonstrates that medical quakery flourished as much in 18th-century Venice as it did in England. Mounted on a platform with his back to us, the charlatan is advertising his medical skill to the gathered crowd. Many of them wear masks and hoods that cover their faces. The wearing of masks may have been an attempt to escape the realities of corrupt 18th-century Venice and also from the thought of death. The charlatan flourished in this type of artificial society. But Tiepolo omits the obvious satire of Hogarth and dwells instead on the more subtle references to decadence implied in the crumbling architecture, the wolf-like masks, the black hoods, and the practitioner of dishonest medicine.

Surgery and Dentistry

In western civilization, the ancestor of the modern surgeon was the barber. Barbers were often the only men who possessed any skill with sharp knives and scissors. They were therefore entrusted with minor, and sometimes even with major, surgical operations. Tonsillectomies, for example, were usually performed by them.

Adriaen Brouwer, whose painting *The Bitter Draught* we have already seen, also painted *The Operation.* The surgeon is undoubtedly a barber, trying his hand at more delicate work. Again, though the interior of the room is rough and simple and the people crude, in Brouwer's hands they become intensely alive.

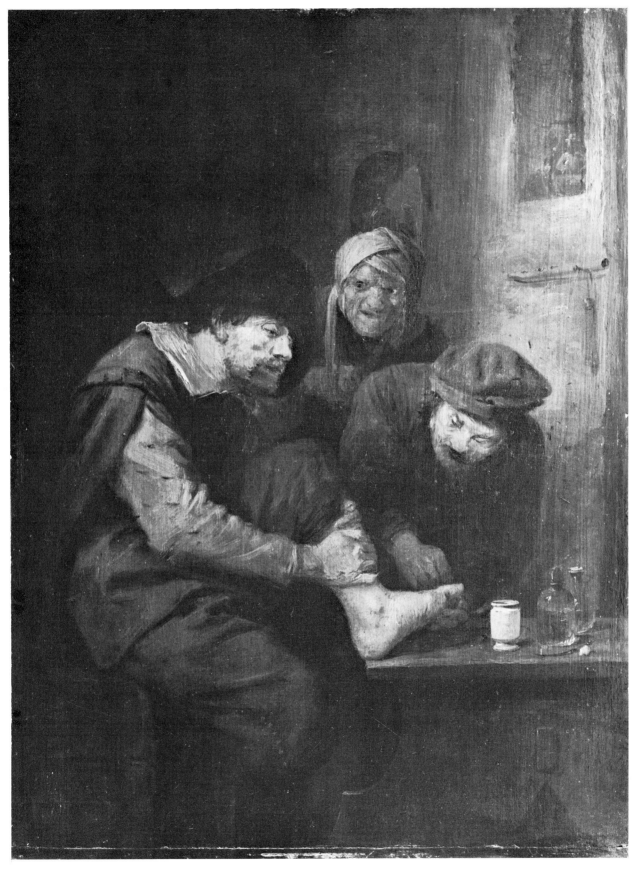

The Operation, by Adriaen Brouwer (1605-1638); Stadel Institute, Frankfurt.

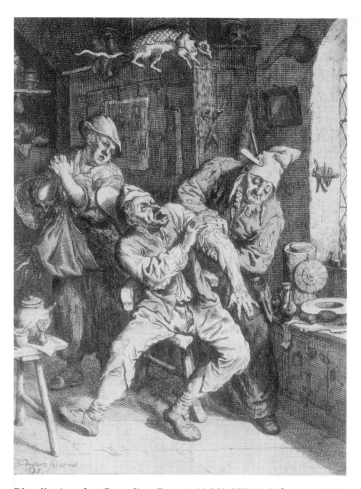

Bloodletting, by Cornelius Dusart (1660-1704); Library of the New York Academy of Medicine.

From ancient times until the 19th century, the practice of opening the veins to release blood was thought to be an effective remedy against disease. The etching *Bloodletting* by the Dutch artist Cornelis Dusart illustrates this widespread practice. An etching is a picture printed from a copper plate on which a drawing has been made with a sharp tool. The lines thus made are etched onto the plate by the use of an acid. Many copies can be made from one etched plate. The technique of etching became widely used after the invention of printing. It is admirably suited to a picture like *Bloodletting*, whose precision and wealth of detail make it an important medical document as well as a work of art.

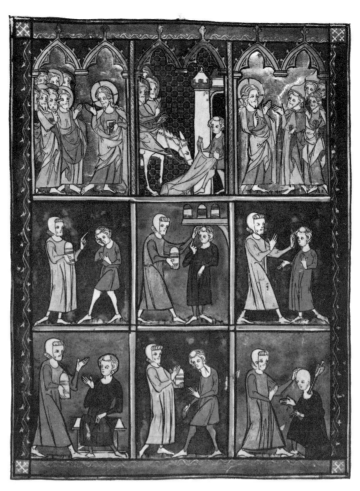

Three Operations, Surgical Manuscript of the School of Salerno (11th century); British Museum, London.

Surgery as it was practiced in the 11th century is vividly illustrated in this page from an illuminated Italian manuscript. Meant as a treatise on various surgical techniques, it included instructions (in Latin) for performing a variety of operations. The colors are bold and the figures flat and decorative. Though the illustrations are unsophisticated by our standards, such manuscripts were an important step toward modern medical knowledge. Considering the lack of hygiene, the use of primitive instruments, and the absence of any anesthetics, it is a wonder that any 11th-century patient ever survived such attempts at a cure.

Operation Scene by William Hogarth, whose *Visit to the Quack Doctor* we have seen, is a quick sketch done in pen and thin ink wash. It depicts a doctor performing surgery on a patient lying in a canopied four-poster bed. You can see that there is an element of satire in the drawing. The exhausted assistant holding the doctor's box of tools almost collapses from fatigue, while the sleepy maidservant holds a candle that is just about to set fire to the doctor's elaborate wig. The patient is almost hidden by the heavy bedclothes — except for one foot sticking out from the blanket. Hogarth loved to play with slender, curving lines, for he maintained that a graceful line was in itself a thing of beauty. This drawing, or rather hasty sketch, was probably intended as a study model for a larger and more finished painting.

Detail from Operation Scene, by William Hogarth (1697-1764); The Pierpont Morgan Library, New York.

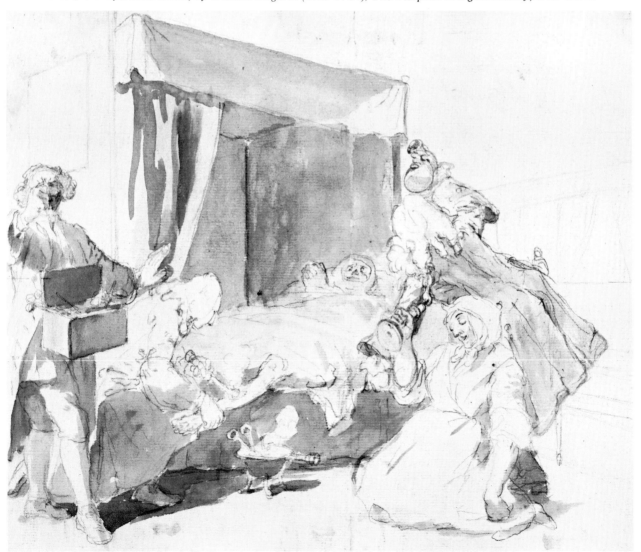

An equally summary sketchiness character-izes the drawing, also called *The Operation*, by Raoul Dufy (dyoo-FEE), a contemporary French painter. At first glance this sketch looks like nothing more than a bunch of squiggly lines, but if you look carefully, you can see that four robed and masked figures are leaning over an operating table intent on the operation that is in progress. A fifth figure stands at a distance behind an instrument table. Like Hogarth, Dufy enjoyed playing with swirling lines that give movement and life to a drawing. With only a few quick strokes of a pen, both artists suggest the drama of the fight against illness and disease.

The Operation, by Raoul Dufy (1877-1953); Musée National d'Art Moderne, Paris.

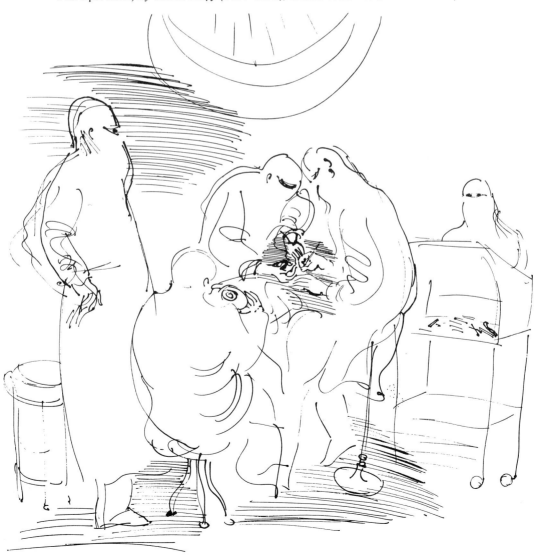

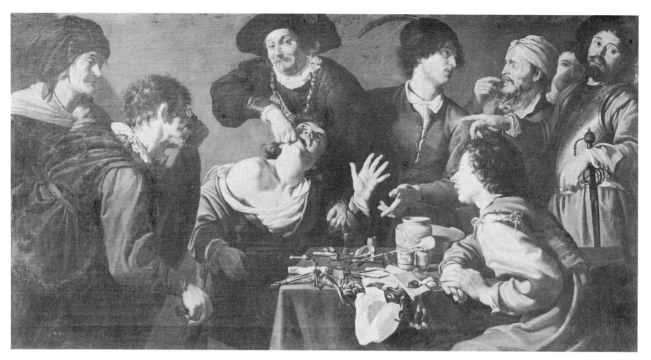

The Tooth Puller, by Theodor Rombouts (1597-1637); Museo del Prado, Madrid.

Dentistry too was practiced on a rather primitive level until fairly recently. Theodor Rombouts, a Flemish painter of the 17th century, leans strongly toward caricature in his painting of *The Tooth Puller*. The figures assume rather exaggerated poses and facial expressions as they watch with both interest and apprehension. Perhaps their turn is coming next. Some of the instruments on the table can be recognized as prototypes of modern dental and medical instruments. A pair of forceps lies in the middle of the table and a crank-turned dental drill in the corner. A strong, harsh light falls on the figures from an unseen source on the left. It creates a strong pattern of light and shadow which heightens the drama of the scene. The central figure, the young man having his tooth extracted, is bathed in the strongest light of all, as if to emphasize his pain. The dentist behind him looks smilingly not at him but out of the picture at us. His attitude makes us grateful that dentistry has progressed a great deal since his day.

Another *Tooth Puller* was depicted by Pietro Longhi (LONG-gea), a Venetian painter of the 18th century. Unlike Rombouts, he does not use strong, dramatic light to heighten reality. Instead his light is subdued and even. But his painting is nevertheless dramatic in another sense: it seems to portray a stage play complete with backdrop and costumed actors. The tooth puller stands on top of a table at stage center, holding up the tooth he has just extracted. His patient (victim, we are tempted to say) sits beneath him holding a handkerchief to his bloody mouth. Other people, including a dwarf, are posed in formal groups as a stage director would arrange his actors. In spite of the bloody subject, there is an air of refinement and elegance that matches the play-acting artificiality of the scene.

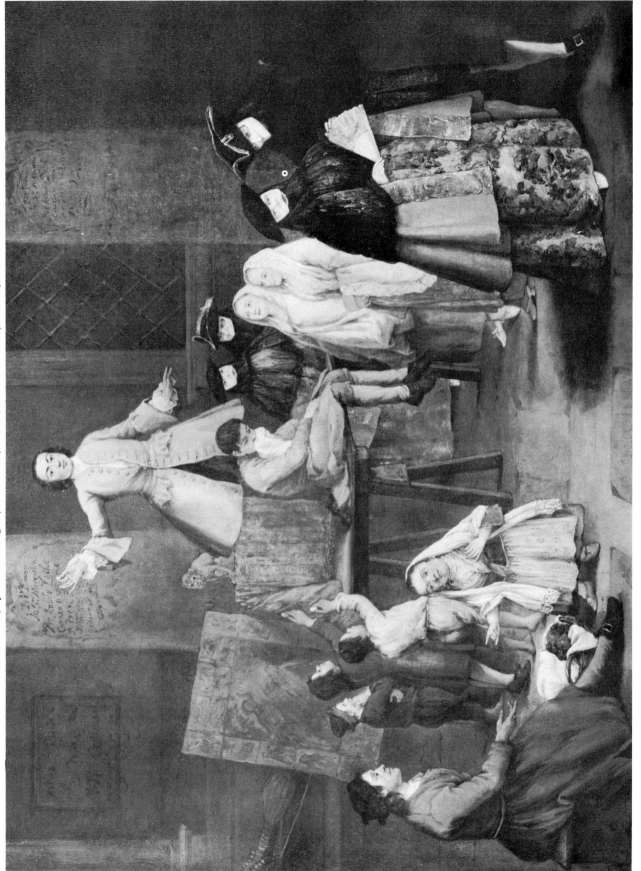

Tooth Puller, by Pietro Longhi (1702-1785); Brera, Milan; Alinari, Art Reference Bureau.

Knowledge of the Human Body Leads to Modern Medicine

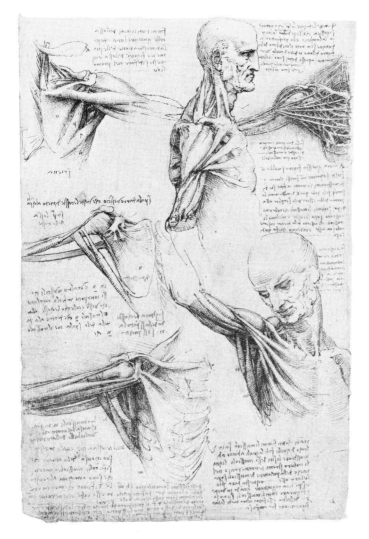

Study of Shoulder and Neck Muscles, by Leonardo da Vinci (1452-1519); Royal Collection, Windsor Castle, Berkshire; reproduced by gracious permission of Her Majesty Queen Elizabeth II.

Much of our knowledge of anatomy we owe to the curiosity and anatomical investigations of artists. They wanted to know exactly how the human body was put together so that they could reproduce its appearance accurately in painting and sculpture. At a time when dissection was frowned on, or even forbidden, they had to carry on their research secretly or at night.

Leonardo da Vinci, whose drawing of an embryo we have already seen, had as pro-found a knowledge of human anatomy as he did of the laws of perspective or the methods of mixing paint. He filled notebook after notebook with beautiful drawings accurate enough to be included in modern anatomical textbooks. Here we see just one of many drawings he made of the muscles of the neck, complete with notes on his own observations. It was from such preliminary studies that he was able to give his painted portraits the feeling of life itself.

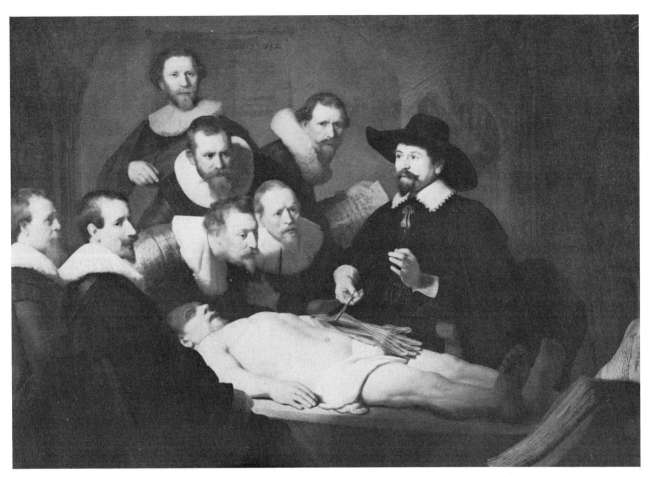

The Anatomy Lesson of Dr. Tulp, by Rembrandt van Rijn (1606-1669); Mauritshuis, The Hague.

Another great artist who carried on his own anatomical investigations was the Dutch painter Rembrandt van Rijn (REM-brant van rhine). In 17th-century Holland, the practice of human dissection was no longer forbidden. Rembrandt shows us an eminent professor of anatomy, Dr. Tulp, lecturing to his pupils over a cadaver that he has just dissected. With a marvelous sense of design, Rembrandt has composed the group of teacher and pupils into a monumental whole in which he nevertheless manages to portray the individual personality of each person. The cadaver stretched out on the table leads our eye inward to the students gathered around it and then up to the professor sitting in his chair. A large, open book serves to close off the composition to the right. The light bathes the living figures in a soft, warm glow that makes us conscious of the transparent atmosphere surrounding them. We feel as though we ourselves are listening to Professor Tulp's anatomy lesson.

Doctors: Divine and Human

Good health was once regarded as a special gift of divine providence and its practitioners were thought of as deities endowed with enormous powers. One such deity was the Egyptian god of good health and medicine, Imhotep. Imhotep may originally have been a real person, a doctor or civil servant who lived around 2600 B.C. Because of his extraordinary skill as a physician, he soon became a legend and was ultimately transformed into the deity of medicine. He is always shown with a shaven head and very often (though not in our illustration) in the company of priests, stressing the close connection in ancient times between the practice of medicine and the priesthood.

Imhotep is carved from a solid block of stone. The folds of his robe are mere lines *incised*, or cut, into the surface of the stone to form a decorative pattern. He holds a scroll which presumably contains prayers and medical recipes.

Imhotep, Egyptian Deity of Medicine; Louvre, Paris; Photograph Giraudon.

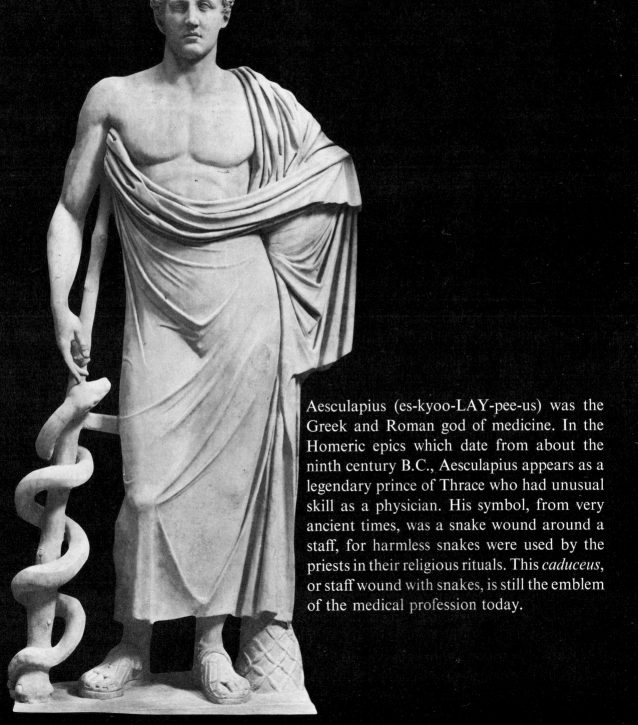

Aesculapius (es-kyoo-LAY-pee-us) was the Greek and Roman god of medicine. In the Homeric epics which date from about the ninth century B.C., Aesculapius appears as a legendary prince of Thrace who had unusual skill as a physician. His symbol, from very ancient times, was a snake wound around a staff, for harmless snakes were used by the priests in their religious rituals. This *caduceus*, or staff wound with snakes, is still the emblem of the medical profession today.

Aesculapius: Vatican Museum, Rome; Alinari, Art Reference Bureau

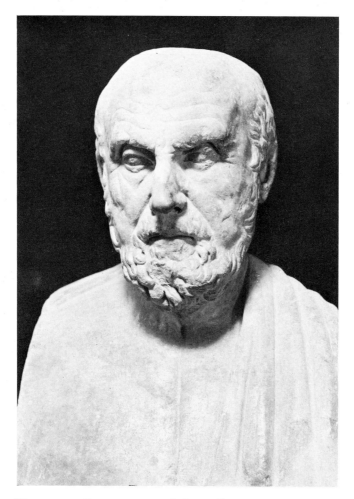

Hippocrates, Roman statue of the Hellenistic period; Vatican Museum, Rome; Alinari, Art Reference Bureau.

Hippocrates, however, was not a legendary figure, but a real physician who was born in Greece around 460 B.C. Called "the father of modern medicine," he was the first to try to separate medicine from magic and to base it instead on natural science and observed fact.

The statue of Hippocrates, like that of Aesculapius, dates from the period of the Roman empire, an era known for its great fondness for portrait sculpture. While the statue of Aesculapius is an idealized one and hardly the portrait of a specific individual, that of Hippocrates seems to be the image of the person portrayed. The art of portrait sculpture in the Roman world has seldom, if ever, been equalled since.

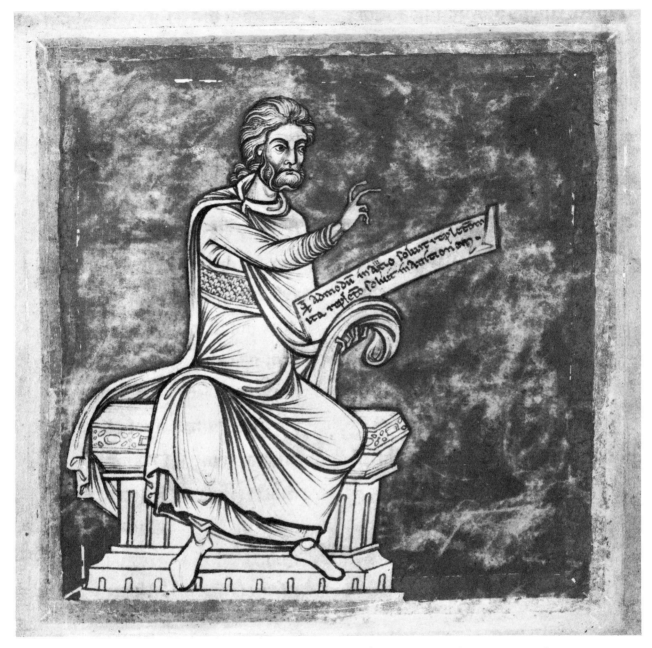

Portrait of a Physician from a medical treatise (11th century); British Museum, London.

This portrait of a physician is from a medical treatise of the 11th century. The portrait is hardly a good likeness of the doctor it is meant to represent. The figure is flat and weightless and the features are indicated in the most general way. The swirling lines of drapery are livelier than the seated figure. In medieval art the drapery often seems to have a life of its own.

Sts. Cosmas and Damian, by Francesco Pesellino (1422-1457); Louvre, Paris; Photograph Giraudon.

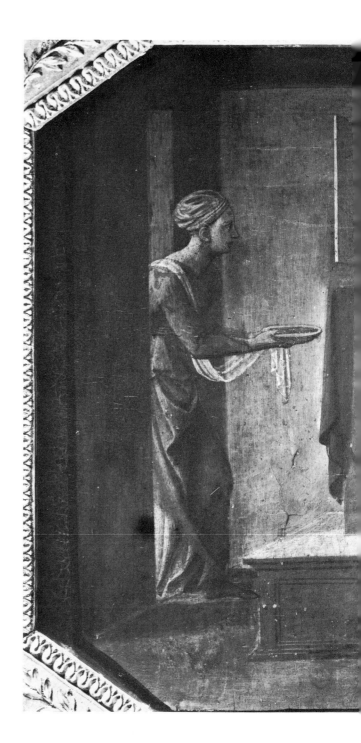

In the Middle Ages the two brothers, Cosmas and Damien, became the patron saints of medical science. They were two early Christian martyrs who, because of their special skill in the medical arts, were frequently shown in paintings with a medical theme. They were specially invoked in times of plague. According to legend, they acquired their reputation by one of the earliest transplants recorded in history—the transplanting of the leg of a Negro to the body of a white man.

Francesco Pesselino (pay-zell-LEE-no), an Italian Renaissance artist, illustrated the two patron saints of medicine in the painting *Sts. Cosmas and Damien.* The doctors, distinguished by their special hats, show sympathy and deep concern as they bend over the sick man lying in bed. The figures are no longer flat and decorative as in the 11th-century treatise, but solid and weighty. We feel their actual presence in the room and the space they occupy. This 15th-century artist has used the new science of perspective and the knowledge of how lines converge in the distance to create the illusion of three-dimensional space on a two-dimensional surface.

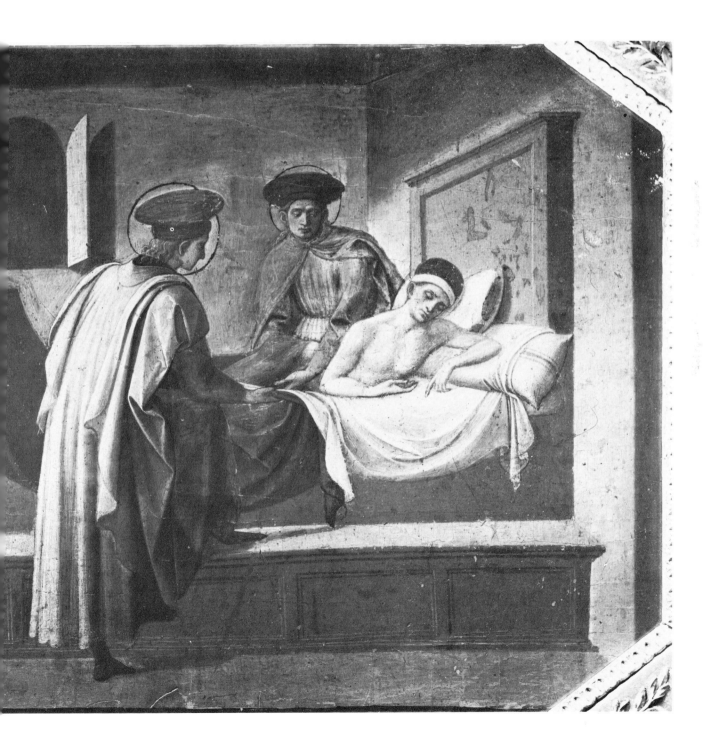

A *Village Doctor* of 17th-century Flanders is shown in a painting by David Teniers the Younger. The theme is one that is familiar to modern medicine — urine analysis — and it indicates how far medical practice had progressed from the superstitious rituals of previous ages. Like Brouwer, Teniers was interested in ordinary people and everyday events, a type of subject matter that we call *genre*. The worried patient standing behind the doctor is a humble soul, and even the doctor is shown without affectation. The soft light shining in through the window picks up the objects whose textures the artist has carefully reproduced — the glass bottles, clay jars, the heavy wooden furniture, and the weighty medical books that are spread open before the doctor. The grave concern of both patient and doctor is vividly shown as well.

Benjamin Rush (1745?-1813) was an American physician, chemist, teacher, and philosopher. He was also an early inquirer into the causes of mental disease and the organizer of the first free medical clinic in the United States.

Village Doctor, by David Teniers the Younger (1610-1690); Palais des Beaux-Arts, Brussels.

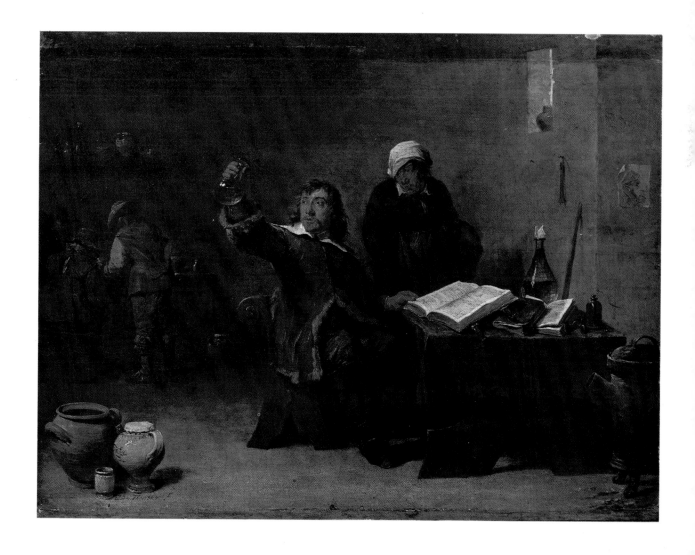

54

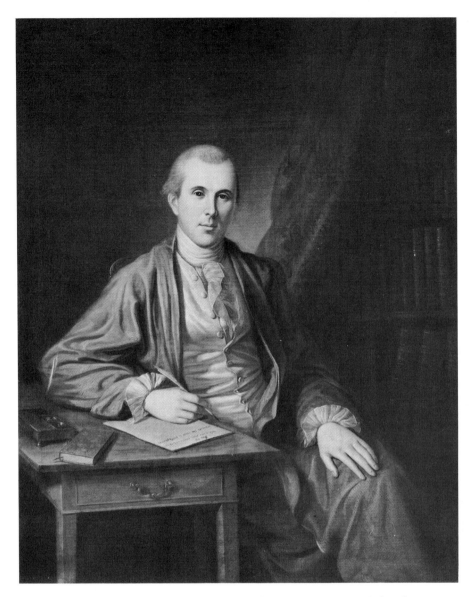

Portrait of Benjamin Rush, by Charles Willson Peale (1741-1827); The Henry Francis du Pont Winterthur Museum, Winterthur; gift of Mrs. T. Charlton Henry.

Rush suggested that the yellow fever epidemics which regularly scourged the eastern seaboard were caused partly by poor sanitation. This theory shocked his fellow Philadelphians and brought him ridicule from the medical profession. His open and inquiring mind, however, and his valuable research, eventually earned him an important place in the history of medicine.

Both Rush and the artist who painted his portrait were good friends of President Thomas Jefferson. The artist, Charles Willson Peale, like Rush, lived in Philadelphia and was interested in science and philosophy as well as art. Peale established one of the first museums in this country and he painted many of the nation's famous men. The portrait of his friend Rush is typical of American painting at the end of the 18th century. It is a simple, direct, and forthright portrait of a distinguished man.

Portrait of Dr. Gachet, by Vincent van Gogh (1853-1890); Mrs. Siegfried Kramarsky, New York.

About a century later, a great Dutch artist, who was himself suffering from mental disease, painted a portrait of his doctor. The portrait of Dr. Gachet is by Vincent van Gogh (van GO). Van Gogh believed that a painting should express an artist's emotions. That is precisely what the portrait of Dr. Gachet does. Using brilliant colors and broad, vigorous brushstrokes, the artist seems to have attacked the canvas as though it were a living opponent. Out of this silent struggle between the artist and the idea he wished to express came a portrait that vibrates with the energy of life yet is subdued by an awareness of human suffering.

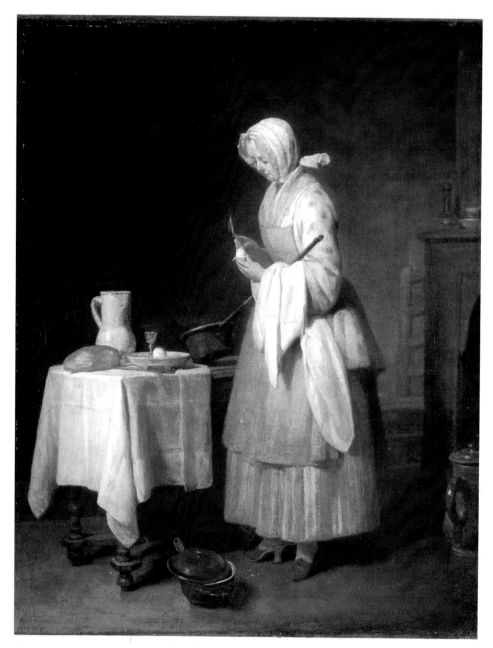

The Attentive Nurse, by Jean Baptiste Simeon Chardin (1699-1779); National Gallery of Art, Washington, D.C.; Samuel H. Kress Collection.

Nurses

Nurses too have been celebrated by artists through the centuries for their devotion to humanity and their tender care of the sick.

The Attentive Nurse was painted by a French artist of the 18th century, Jean Baptiste Simeon Chardin (shar-DAN). Like the Dutch masters Brouwer and Teniers, Chardin liked to paint ordinary people engaged in simple tasks. Yet so great was his skill in arranging the people and objects he saw into balanced, harmonious compositions, that they lose their everyday quality and acquire the soft rhythms of poetry or quiet music.

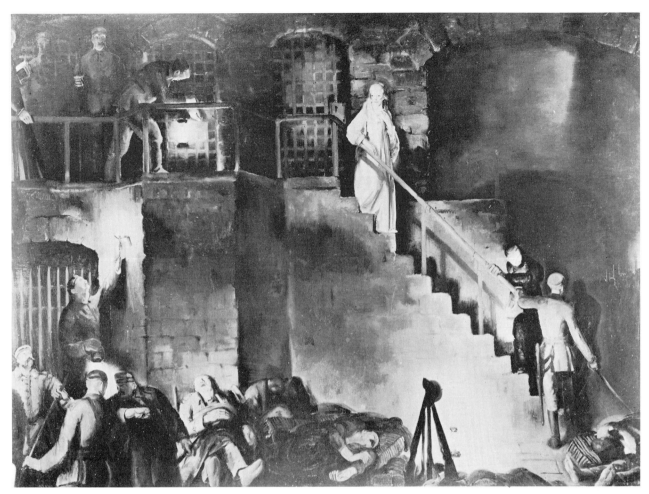

Edith Cavell (1918), by George Wesley Bellows (1882-1925); Museum of Fine Arts, Springfield; James Philip Gray Collection.

Edith Cavell was an army nurse for the Allied forces during World War I. She was captured by the Germans who accused her of being a spy and then shot her. Her execution aroused much indignation, and the courage with which she met her death won her world-wide admiration. Her story fired the imagination of the American painter, George Bellows, who painted her in the hands of her German captors on the way to prison and death. It is a dramatic conception of this brave nurse, almost as though, like the Venetian, Longhi, Bellows were visualizing a stage production. The heroine is at stage center, the villians surround her, and the light flickers fitfully on the prison walls.

Night Duty, by Franklin Boggs (1914-   ); United States Army Historical Collection, Washington, D.C.

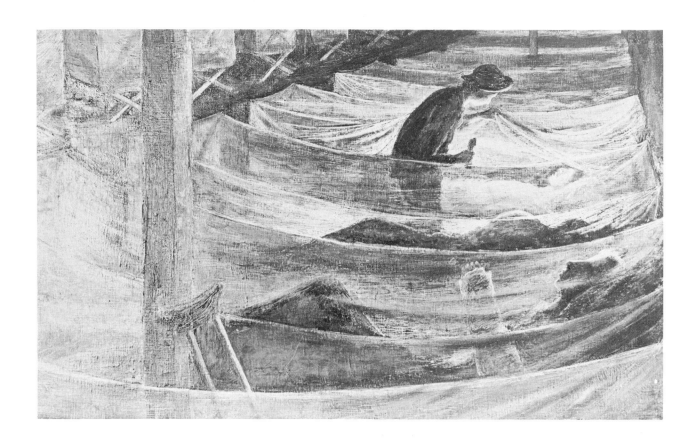

The nurse in Franklin Boggs's *Night Duty* is a much more anonymous person than Edith Cavell and a less dramatic one. But though we do not know her name, her obvious dedication to nursing and steady devotion to her patients make her just as much a heroine. She is an American army nurse of World War II, shown as she makes her night rounds administering to the wounded soldiers in her care. As she lifts the mosquito netting over one wounded soldier and bends to look at him, the glow from the small flashlight illuminates her averted face and sharply patterns the rows of hammocks in the hospital ward. Though Boggs creates a much more abstract composition than does Bellows, his painting is just as forceful in underlining the steady heroism that is so much a part of a nurse's profession.

Hospitals and Clinics

Although early hospitals were meant to help the sick and to relieve their suffering, their lack of the simplest sanitary arrangements and their overcrowding made many of them merely a prelude to death.

As the *miniature*, or illustration, from a 14th-century French illuminated manuscript shows, frequently two or more patients suffering from various diseases were placed in the same bed. The patients in this picture are attended by nuns who often did, and still do,

make nursing their religious duty. Some of the figures are larger than others in order to emphasize their importance. Though the unknown artist had difficulty with perspective, there is no mistaking the misery of the sick people lying in the beds. His miniature is an important historical document of the primitive conditions which made people in ages past fear commitment to a hospital as much as death itself.

Sick Ward at Hotel Dieu (15th century); Musée de l' Assistance Publique, Paris; Photograph Giraudon.

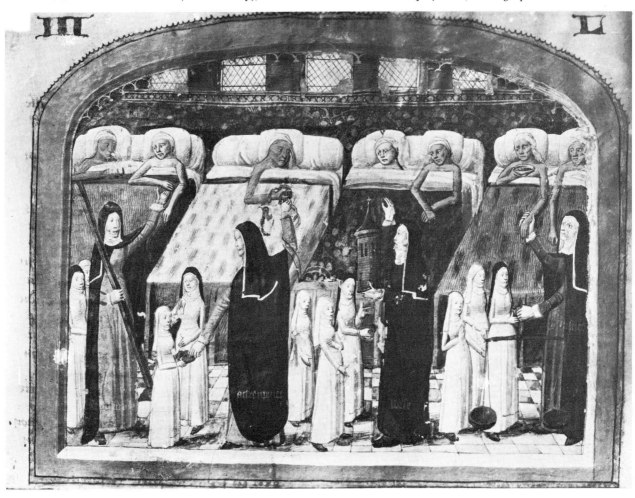

Hospital conditions had improved somewhat by the 18th century. A print of a hospital in Middlesex, England, by Thomas Rowlandson shows that now, at least, only one patient to a bed was the rule and some small effort was made toward cleanliness. Of course this was still very far from the antiseptic conditions of the modern hospital. The curtains around one of the beds indicate a growing awareness of the need for privacy and dignity even when a person is ill or in pain.

Hospital—Middlesex, by Thomas Rowlandson (1756-1827); Museum of Fine Arts, Springfield; gift of Homans Robinson.

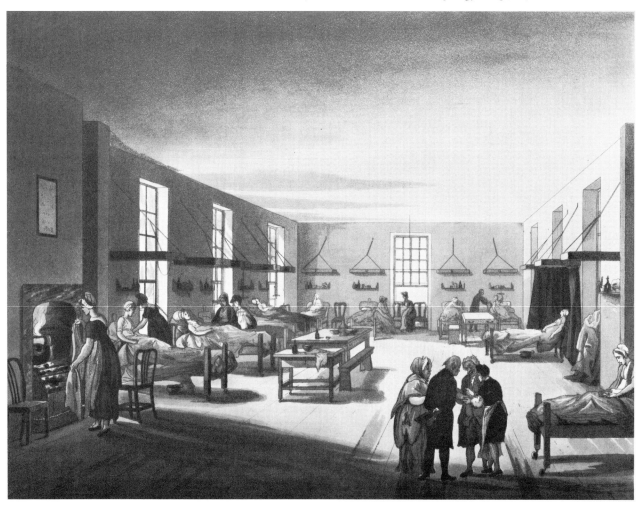

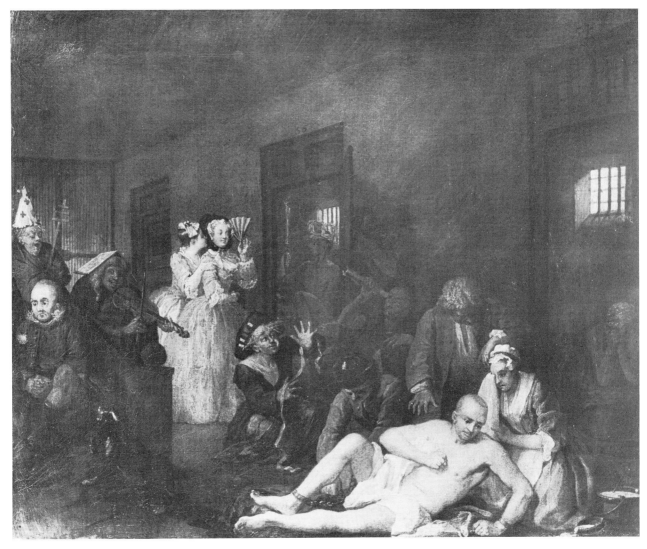

A Visit to Bedlam (The Mad House), by William Hogarth (1697-1764); Sir John Soane's Museum, London.

In 18th-century mental hospitals, however, conditions were not only primitive, but they showed a complete lack of understanding of the nature of mental disease. This ignorance is evident in William Hogarth's painting, *A Visit to Bedlam*. Bedlam, a contraction of the name Bethlehem, was originally the hospital of St. Mary of Bethlehem, founded in London in the 13th century. In time it was given over to the care of the insane and the word "bedlam" indicates the kind of care they received. The patients were chained and manacled or merely left to their sick delusions, while society ladies, dressed up in their finery, came to laugh at them as part of an afternoon's entertainment. Hogarth was many years ahead of his time in criticizing the terrible conditions of the mental hospitals of his time.

In order to celebrate the bravery of his emperor, a French painter of the early 19th century portrayed *Napoleon Visiting the Plague Patients at Jaffa*. The picture illustrates an incident in one of Napoleon's Middle Eastern campaigns, and though the artist, Antoine Jean Gros (an-twann zhahn grow), was more attracted by the color and exotic flavor of an oriental scene than by medical conditions in Palestine in 1799, he nevertheless left a vivid picture of a hospital for plague patients at that time.

Two famous paintings by an American artist, Thomas Eakins (AY-kinz), illustrate the great advances made in medical science and hospital techniques during the second half of the 19th century. The first one, The Gross Clinic (frontispiece), was painted in 1875 and shows Dr. Samuel David Gross in his clinic at Jefferson Medical College in Philadelphia. Dr. Gross was one of the greatest surgeons, teachers, and writers on surgery that the United States has produced. With scalpel in hand he talks to his students during an operation he is performing. His intelligent face, framed by a mass of bushy white hair, dominates the scene. There is a sense of reality, of closeness to the subject, that may recall Rembrandt's *Anatomy Lesson of Dr. Tulp*. In Rembrandt's painting, of course, the lecture was over a cadaver and lacked the drama and sense of tension that a living patient provides in Eakins's painting.

Napoleon Visiting the Plague Patients at Jaffa, by A. J. Gros (1771-1835); Louvre, Paris; Photograph Giraudon.

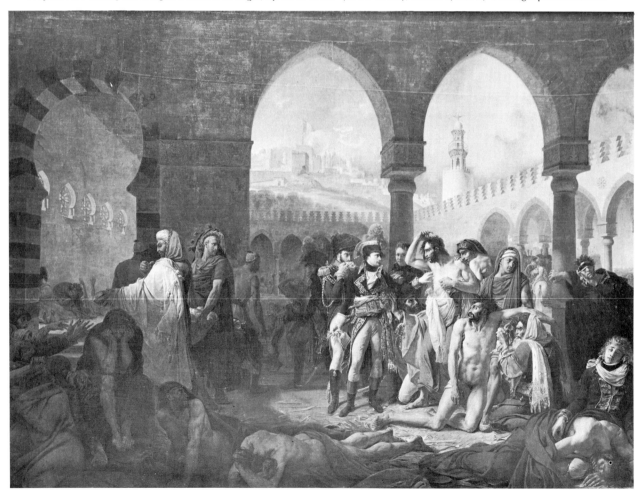

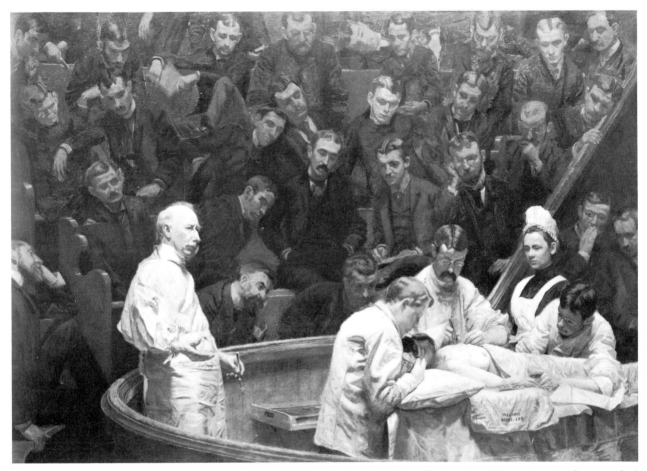

The Agnew Clinic (1889), by Thomas Eakins (1844-1916); School of Medicine, University of Pennsylvania; photographed by The Philadelphia Museum of Art.

Fourteen years later, in 1889, Eakins painted another picture of an eminent surgeon in his clinic. *The Agnew Clinic* portrays Dr. D. Hayes Agnew, a professor at the Medical School of the University of Pennsylvania. If you compare the paintings of the two clinics, you will see how conditions had changed since 1875. The new knowledge of asepsis and its application in medical practice is illustrated in the sterile white gowns and rubber gloves that Dr. Agnew and his assistants wear. The anesthetist holds an ether cone over the patient's nose rather than smothering him with an anesthetic-soaked cloth as in the earlier painting. No longer are the patients' relatives allowed into the operating theatre. By the beginning of the 20th century, medical practice had become a modern profession performed by highly trained and competent practitioners. After many centuries of trial and error, of the gradual synthesis of observed fact, of brilliant guesses and groping experiments, medicine had become a truly healing art.

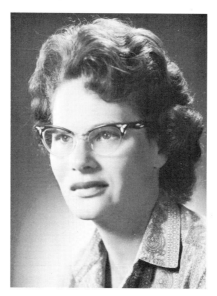

the author

Rena Neumann Coen is an assistant professor of art history at St. Cloud State College in St. Cloud, Minnesota. She has been a research assistant at the Minneapolis Institute of Arts, and her articles on art history have appeared in several art publications. She is the author of *Kings and Queens in Art*, *American History in Art*, *The Black Man in Art*, and *The Old Testament in Art*.

Mrs. Coen is a native of New York City. She earned her B.A. degree at Barnard College, her M.A. at Yale University, and her Ph.D. at the University of Minnesota. She is the wife of Professor Edward Coen of the Department of Economics at the University of Minnesota. The Coens and their three children live in Minneapolis.

the designer

Patricia Koskey studied art at the University of Minnesota, Duluth, and at the School of Associated Arts in St. Paul, Minnesota, where she teaches classes in design. She worked as a staff artist on the *Duluth Herald and News-Tribune* before entering the field of book design. In her spare time, Miss Koskey enjoys designing and making humorous greeting cards.